Healthy Living Habits

Healthy Living Habits

How To Start Eating Mindfully, Living Longer, and Feeling Better Every Day

Dominque Kaneza

Table of Contents:

Chapter 1
What is meant by healthy eating?

All things considered, talking about food is probably the next best thing to eating. When you think of food, if the first thing that takes shape in your head is the image of a nice juicy steak or a hamburger, then probably it is the time to reconsider your eating habits. More importantly, if you are responsible for family meals, then spending some time getting to know the right foods to eat, cook and serve will set you off along the right path to healthy eating.

Mayo Clinic has reported that middle-aged American men who eat heartily are at a far greater risk for chronic heart diseases than their counterparts in countries like Greece. The root of the problem as per the study lies in poor diet and lack of exercise.

This problem has multiplied over the years to become a national health issue. Respected American institution like the AHA and ACSM, in their initiative to promote awareness about health, have urged the nation to educate themselves about their diet.

Should I re-evaluate my eating habits?

"Health is Wealth" is a saying that speaks for itself. Healthy eating does not mean you change your lifestyle as an immediate measure. Neither does it mean that you place yourself on a diet. Your eating habits are a reflection of your emotional and mental state. Lucille Ball very aptly said that "*the secret of staying young is to live honestly, eat slowly and lie about your age.*" We know this popular actress as someone who also took good care of her health. There is a world of good advice in there when you think about it. Chewing the food well *does* help you digest your food and when you live within your means, it *does* reduce the stress!

The idea is to not disown your likes and dislikes, but work toward making subtle changes to your diet to improve your energy levels, so as to enable your body to perform the daily schedule of activities with little or no stress. For example; taking sufficient calcium is absolutely necessary as you grow older especially for women who are at risk for osteoporosis.

"The secret of success in life is to eat what you like and let the food fight it out inside" said the great American Humorist Mark Twain, more than a hundred years ago. Humor aside, as you get older, what you eat on a regular basis is the battle that is to be fought. You need to become more particular about the *portions* you eat of the things you like the most.

Be your own hero – discover what works for you

Many books have been written on what constitutes the perfect diet. Advice upon advice has been sent your way by the experts on nutrition. As a layman, your confusion is not surprising. Educating yourself about food groups and taking a good hard look at the food triangle would be your first goal.

At the base of the food triangle lie the whole grains, fresh fruits, nuts and vegetables. These food groups are made up of carbohydrate, fiber, fat and nutrients essential for the body. It should form the basis of your diet making up about 70 percent of the food on your plate. The rest of the 30 percent should be proteins and dairy. If you are a diabetic, increasing the quantity of fiber will provide bulk and help you suppress the hunger pangs.

Be a super hero and start reading labels before you buy. Check for the presence of saturated and unsaturated fats and unhealthy preservatives. Every food package has to provide a list of nutrients and chemicals present in its contents

As you transition to a healthier lifestyle, make a list of changes that will help lessen your intake of unhealthy foods. Cut back on the fatty cholesterols by reaching for olive oil instead of butter at the grocery. Replace polished rice with whole grains so that you do not lose the nutrients. Use a non-stick frying pan; it allows you to cook with less oil.

Free yourself from the burden of eating processed food by enjoying a cooked meal from your own kitchen. It gives you the freedom to pick and choose the ingredients for the dishes you make!

The better the quality of the foods you eat, the greater is the feeling of well being. Your immunity rises, as does your energy levels helping you to perform better days after days and years after years.

Peer pressure – finding it hard to say no to gooey desserts

If you feel pressure in having to skip all the things you love eating in your effort to switch over to healthy eating, then pause to consider your feelings. After all, you are doing this for yourself and your family. When you do something and feel bad afterwards, then your efforts may be in vein making you crash out.

It is a better idea to change slowly. Enjoy your sweet desserts and beverages; but take them in smaller quantity and less often. Next time you go out for tea at the cake shop, order a muffin or share your slice of the truffle with a friend. Even better, pack half to enjoy later.

The less sugar, salt and butter you give to your body, the smoother will be the blood flow in your veins and the less will be the pressure on your heart. If you have a sweet tooth, try adding sweet vegetables like yam and onions to your dishes to reduce cravings for desserts. When you brew tea and coffee lightly, they do not taste bitter and you get to savor their fragrance and flavor without having to add sugar.

Less is more as far as salt and health is concerned. If you must have your food salty, try adding some lemon juice, which is naturally salty and flavorful, directly to your food when you sit down to eat.

Moderation is the way to healthy eating, whether that is the cup of the vintage rouge or the portion of the rare flank on your plate.

Eating in good company – learning to swim in uncharted waters

Food is the spice of life; but when you add conversation, the simplest dishes turn special. You talk and eat slowly allowing yourself to savor the foods you are eating and drinking. While for many, it may be the most natural way to eat in company, for many others it requires to be inculcated. This is very helpful when you make a transition to eating healthy with like-minded people. You eat as much or as little as you want focusing on interaction with others. Your attention shifts from the food to the ambiance and the essence of the food and how you eat it.

This is a great way to enjoy food from other cultures. Opening your mind to new foods and learning to make them in your own kitchen widens your food network with healthy dishes that can become popular amongst family and friends.

For many, eating foods from a different culture may not sound palatable. If you are adventurous try eating out with a knowledgeable friend to explore dishes that suit your taste buds. If you are a hack at fried foods, try steamed cuisine recipes, which are equally delicious and a lot healthier.

If you are not a great fan of cooking; but would not mind trying to inculcate the habit, you can make a good start by asking friends to join you in the kitchen and helping you make a meal. Try simple dishes avoiding elaborate meals.

Feel good eating – pick up a bar of chocolate

If you are feeling overwhelmed at the thought of healthy eating turning into an era of deprivation, you could be proved wrong. Consider replacing the rich chocolate cake with a bar of chocolate and enjoying a piece whenever you want to. That would be a great way to make a transition to a healthier lifestyle and keep the endorphins going while your heart remains ship-shape!

It is a well established fact that when you reduce your daily sugar intake via your teas and coffees to zero, your cravings for sweet desserts and drinks diminish over time. You will ultimately receive equal amounts of satisfaction from smaller servings of these items.

Deprivation is a state of the mind and a body that has been indulged over a long period of time by unwholesome foods. The trick is to replace these unhealthy foods with their leaner, less oily and less sugary smart counterparts.

Search for like-minded people and exchange healthy recipes and tips on good cooking and eating habits. It generates interest and keeps you focused on inculcating healthy eating habits.

"People who love to eat are always the best people" – **Julia Childs**

Many studies have been done to analyze the eating habits of different demographic groups in America for the purpose of managing their *eating disorders*. The bottom line to eating well is to listen to your body and choose the foods, which you yearn for. If the yearning is for junk food, plant little time bombs in your head about their long term health effects and substitute them with well-made tasty and healthy dishes in your own kitchen.

"*A balanced diet is a cookie in each hand*" said American literary critique and Guggenheim Award winning author, Barbara Johnson. While there may be oodles of truism to this quote urging you to think about eating well without stressing over what is on your plate; it is also true that in order to lead a healthy and vital life, you have to learn to say *no* to junk food and inculcate habits that will help you make the right choice of foods. Physical and mental wellness is not a myth, it is a reality, which you may cherish by eating healthy and living well!

Chapter 2
Positive and negative psychological effects of our eating habits

Many parents teach their children from a young age, how to eat well and live a healthy life. Yet, nowadays it is very easily forgotten and maintaining a well-balanced diet is hard.

However, whenever you want to lose weight or get in shape; healthy eating habits provide numerous benefits. In this chapter, we are going to discuss the psychological benefits of eating well as well as the negative impact of dieting.

Relation between diet and mental health

Diet plays a very important role in mental and physical health, and good nutrition is always essential for a healthy mind and body. The food we take contributes a lot in the development, management and prevention of mental conditions like – depression, Alzheimer's disease, schizophrenia, attention deficit hyperactivity disorder, etc. According to a survey conducted by a group of researchers in the UK, people who eat fresh fruits and vegetables on a regular basis have less or no complaints of the above mental problems. Diet that is rich in proteins, vitamins, minerals and adequate amount of carbohydrates can help to balance the moods and feelings and ensure a healthy mind. Diet can even help in the recovery of mental health. For this reason, doctors advise to have a well-balanced diet along with other treatments.

What are the positive effects of a well balanced diet on mind?

Diet and exercise are the two important things that can improve mental health and has shown positive effects on mind. Regular exercise and healthy diet can protect the brain cells and keep you away from mental disorders. There are a number of foods that affect the brain positively as well as negatively. What you put into your body not only affects your body; but also produces an impact on the overall psychological well-being. Foods influence your mood to a great extent and hence, it is essential to make healthy food choices that result in significant improvement in the overall mental and physical health. Below are some of the benefits of eating healthy –

- **Reduces symptoms of mental disorders**

Eating healthy has shown to produce a significant improvement in the mental state. It can reduce the symptoms of depression, bipolar disorder, anxiety, anger and frustration. Eating healthy meals balance the blood sugar levels, which is very essential to balance the mood-swings associated with depression and anxiety. A healthy diet is always free from sugar and related elements to keep the sugar-induced spikes under control.

- **Increases energy levels**

Eating healthy can boost your energy levels and help you feel better about yourself. Unhealthy foods that are rich in sugar or highly processed increase the energy levels significantly; but you will notice a dip immediately after the spike. Due to this, you will feel short burst of energy followed by profound fatigue.

• Keeps brain sharp and alert

Healthy eating habits keep your brain sharp and active all the times. A well-balanced and healthy diet can keep your brain functioning to its optimum level and also enhance your memory. People who include extra virgin olive oil, spinach, apples and grape juice in their regular diet have noticed significant decrease in the symptoms of psychological conditions like – depression, anxiety, anger, frustration, etc.

• Increases confidence levels

Choosing right and healthy food items will control your thoughts and allow you to feel proud. Healthy food choices can induce weight loss and increase positive feelings about self. Your changed appearance can instill confidence in you and improve your self-esteem.

Foods that improve mental health

Mental health professionals say that good eating habits are essential for people who want to optimize their effectiveness and cope up with the negative effects of mental illnesses. It is essential to select food items that have consequences beyond the taste bud satisfaction. You need to have a balanced diet of –

- Fresh fruits and vegetables
- Protein rich food
- Food items that are rich in omega-3 fatty acids
- Whole grains and cereals

Try to include less sugary foods and more wholegrain cereals, beans, nuts, lentils, fruits, vegetables, etc. Whole grains and fruits are more filling, as the sugar in these foods is absorbed slowly. Eat at least 3-4 meals a day to balance the blood sugar levels. Skipping breakfast or meals lowers blood sugar levels significantly and results in low mood, fatigue and irritation. Always try to choose food items like –

1. Bran cereals, wholegrain meal, oats, porridge, etc. which are rich in fiber and low in sugar.
2. Whole meal or granary bread, rye breads, whole meal bread, rice cakes, corn cakes, whole meal chapattis, etc. which are right in carbohydrates and other nutrients.

3. If you love potatoes, serve boiled potatoes with their skins. You may also try sweet potatoes or yams for a change.

4. Have at least 5 portions of fruits and vegetables every day. Tomatoes, bananas and mushroom contain high levels of potassium, which is very essential for a healthy nervous system.

5. Include at least one portion of protein such as – fish, eggs, milk, cheese, nuts, lentils, beans, meat substitute, textured vegetables, etc. at each meal.

6. To make your diet interesting and healthy, eat a wide range of food items. This will not only satisfy your taste buds, but also ensure that you obtain all the essential nutrients.

7. Maintain a healthy weight. Weight is one of the important factors that affect your overall mental health.

8. Maintain adequate intake of water and other fluids. Make sure that you are having least 8-10 glasses of water every day. Depression, mood-swings, anger, negative behavior and thoughts are the early effects of dehydration. So, always stay hydrated by having enough fluid. Try to limit intake of coffee and colas as that contain caffeine that encourages the production of urine and dehydrates the body.

Negative effects of dieting

Till now, you read about the benefits of healthy diet and how it keeps your brain strong and sharp. In this section, you will get answers to questions like –

- Is it really important to eat healthy?
- What happens if you don't follow a balanced diet?
- How dieting affects your mind?

Many people engage in dieting and related activities and keep their body in starvation mode. The popularity of dieting has been fuelled by the most common factor called obesity. The second reason behind dieting is the slimming industry that created a myth that body fat can be controlled by right diet. As far as dieting is concerned, there are some psychological effects, which everyone should understand. Below is the detailed description of psychological effects of dieting –

1. Depression and anxiety

Researchers found that people who do dieting are more likely to experience depressive disorders than those who don't follow dieting practice. Nutrients play a very important role in keeping your brain healthy and women who diet are likely to experience depression, anxiety and even irregular menses.

2. Low self-esteem

People who are on diet are more likely to experience low self-esteem due to their poor body image. Poor body image is the result of either overeating or dieting. You need to aim for a balanced diet and perceive yourself to improve appetite and have a good body structure.

3. Stress

People who are on diet are likely to experience high levels of emotional stress than people who don't diet regularly. Eating a few carbohydrates can increase the stress levels significantly.

4. Mood changes and fatigue

This is the first and foremost symptoms that dieters experience often. Their mood tends to change with the decreasing energy levels. As your body have less food to convert into energy, the blood sugar levels drop and result in irritability, fatigue and even food cravings.

5. Reduced metabolism

The metabolism of your body slows down to conserve some energy while you are on dieting. This will result in loss of muscle tone and weight loss.

Dieting creates an oppressed feeling and leads to stress and irritation. People tend to become more anxious and depressed and find it difficult to concentrate. They tend to stay away from people and experience critical evaluations of their body. At the end of dieting period, the personality of the person is revered to normal state.

The bottom line is – it is essential to have a healthy and well-balanced diet. There is no doubt that dieting is a good practice as it gives rest to the digestive system and cleans the body. However, seeing the negative consequences of dieting on mind, we can say that it is not good to keep your body in "starvation mode" for long period.

Though you are on dieting, you should try to fulfill the minimum nutritional requirements of your body by having adequate amount water, fresh fruit juices, vegetable salads, etc. This will ensure that your body and mind will get sufficient nutrients, especially when you are dieting.

Chapter 3
The list of foods you must avoid

All living beings eat food mostly out of instinct. Food is needed to nourish our body and keep it going. But it is also needed to give us our daily minimum quota of innocent pleasure. Hence, we don't just eat food, we also taste it! It keeps us happily busy for a lot of time, not just while eating it; but also while preparing it or thinking about it with pulsating anticipation. I know many people who start discussing the menu of their dinner even before finishing their lunch. All such generalizations may not be true; but it's a known fact that a way to people's heart is often through their stomach.

Nothing is perfect

However, all good things have their limitations. Foods have many. Even if you feel that this particular food is yummy, you cannot live on it entirely. Your body needs a regular, balanced diet. That means what you eat has to be a varied mixed fare. It has to have all the vitamins, carbohydrates, amino acids, good fats, proteins and the minerals that the body cannot do without. So we must eat a balanced mix of food. We must have the right diet. And some foods are not good for the body. Unfortunately, it happens too often that what you like the most tops the "No No" list of the foods for our body.

O small mercies

The good-diet fanatics are not satisfied with cutting down on all the good food. They have to outdo themselves by admonishing us poor people against eating too much of sugar. And their "too much" is "too little." They blame many ills of the body on sugar and ask us to cut down on candies, chocolates, soft drinks, sweets and deserts.

Then the balanced-diet gangs zoom down on our cigarettes and a peg or two or three a day of liquor. They do not know how difficult our life is. How crucial it is for us to relax. They do not realize that we get huge relief from our daily quota of cigarettes and the pegs. They do not allow us to have the luxury of floating weightlessly in rarified atmosphere after our third peg. Nor do they allow us to chill out with a few beers or wine. They wish to burn down our smoking dreams. We fail to understand why we must forsake these pleasures when they are bringing to us so much of joy and satisfaction. This is nothing short of cruelty. They are depriving us of our small mercies.

Without health, what is life?

But a fact is a fact, is a fact, is a fact!!! A human life is long. The young body of a growing person can take up a lot of unnecessary load and not complain for quite some time. But then, it has its limits. It cannot be overloaded forever. There comes a time and pretty soon too, that the body starts creaking. It starts complaining. Each organ in the body starts giving trouble. We have never been aware of so many organs, body parts or systems in our body. Now each day, yet another new organ sends an "unwell" notice. Soon we realize that a life with so many troubles over such long-drawn years of middle age and old age is not what we wished or deserved. The joyous eating sprees of youth cannot compensate for the pain in every cell of the body in later years. We have to find a way to keep the body hale and hearty right up to the ripe old age.

You must have an all-round healthy diet to lead a long and healthy life. And you also have to keep away from many interesting foods to ensure that you remain fit as a fiddle till an advanced age. This is the reason that we earlier called "cruelty", rather a very valid reason, for the experts to advise you to sacrifice the small pleasures of our life by giving up sweets, alcohol and smoking, so that the life becomes a healthy pleasure later! The list of the foods you must avoid is long. Here are some of them.

The first and the most important ones: Fats and sugars

The body cannot handle too much of saturated fats. That means; you have to drastically cut down on almost all of the whole milk dairy products and red meat. Dairy milk products go into the preparation of many of our favorite dishes, including butter and sweets. And red meat is the daily staple food used in most mouth-watering dishes.

You also have to cut down on trans fats. Margarines, cookies, snacks, candies, fried foods, foods using vegetable oils and baked goods are full of trans fats. And the best way to avoid them is to not prepare them or buy them at all. If you cannot eat cookies, fried foods and snacks to your heart's content, why waste your precious time and energy on preparing them?

And there are a few others as given below:

- Keep miles away from packaged and processed foods such as canned soups and frozen dinners.
- Remember that low-fat meals usually have hidden salt and sugar above the allowable limits. Use fresh vegetables and prepare your meals at home as far as possible.
- Most fast food and restaurant meals have a lot of sodium. Most gravies, dressings and sauces contain extra salt and sugar. Avoid them.
- Reject sweets like candies, chocolates and cakes. Replace them with fruits.
- Study labels and select products with low sodium and sugar.
- No sugary drinks please. Try sparkling water with fruit juice.
- Microwave popcorn packed in bags contains many harmful chemicals. Do not try them.
- Stick margarine is full of trans-fats. They mean calories, 100 in each tablespoon. They damage

your blood vessels and arteries. Real butter will be a better idea, if used in moderation.

- Pancakes made of pancake mix have hydrogenated soybean or cottonseed oil. This means a lot of trans fat. They also have preservatives and salt. Make pancakes from your own mix.
- Shun artificial sweeteners. They rid the body of its ability to know how much it has consumed. That results in your overeating. The artificial sweeteners persuade you to eat more sweets. Diet sodas double the risk of you gaining extra weight.
- Tomatoes are good, not tomato sauce or ketchup. It has corn syrup or sugar. It also has sodium. Fresh home-made tomato sauce is healthier and cheaper. The artificial colors, flavors and preservatives of commercial sauce make them worse.
- Canned frosting contains trans-fats, corn syrup, preservatives, artificial colors and flavors. Do not even try it.
- Packaged sandwiches have white bread and mayonnaise. That means; too much of fat and salt intake. Cheese adds to the fat content. The meat used is unhealthy. It could also be left over from the earlier day. A sandwich has over 400 calories. Enough reasons to not even think of them.

- Coleslaw contains good cabbage and carrot. But their good is more than neutralized by the sugars and fat coming from mayonnaise. Better to make your own Coleslaw at home with yogurt.

- The warm moist conditions in which sprouts grow are good for bacteria too. Sprouts give you no idea how old they are. Sprouts with bacteria can be dangerous.

- A slice of marketed pizza has the salt content enough to make up the four days' requirement for any person, depending upon the topping. Salt, cheese and sausage in the pizza spell too many nitrates. Its palm oil, sugar and fats add to the calories. You have an excellent alternative: a home-made pizza.

- If you start eating salty snacks, you keep eating them. Don't start.

- Ranch dressing is put on burgers, fries and pizzas. It tastes great. But each tablespoon has 75 calories and 7 grams of fat. It also has sugar, food starch, artificial flavors and colors. You do not want these in your body.

- Fast foods are full of trans fats, salt, chemicals and sugars. The special burgers have more than 19 grams of saturated fats. A serving of French fries has 4 days' worth of trans fat. Do not even think of fast foods.

Good food is tasty too

You must be careful about what you eat all the time. More so when you are eating out or eating packaged food. The list of foods to be avoided keeps growing. One may think why and how can we eat only bland food all the time? This is not true. Healthy food can be tasty. You only have to try and make it. And you do not have to abstain from the "banned" food all the time. Our body is a miraculous device. If we recognize its capacities and remain well within its limits, it will allow you to occasionally have a go at the prohibited foods.

The key to eating well and maintaining the body is moderation. A famous actor who was active until his 90s used to say, "I never eat food. I just taste it." Follow the moderation guru, taste everything; but in small measure and you will be all right!

Chapter 4
Lifestyle habits that facilitate or hinder healthy eating

By hearing the term 'healthy eating', people often think it as something with strict dietary limitations. Rather, it is about feeling great, stabilizing your mood and improving your outlook. Remember that you are not the only person who is overwhelmed by the conflicting diet advice. You will find lots of experts who tell that certain food is good for you. On the contrary, you will find people who say exactly opposite and tell that the same food is not good.

Your lifestyle and habits will have a great impact on your eating habits and overall health. In this chapter, we are going to discuss a few lifestyle habits that facilitate or hinder healthy eating.

Lifestyle habits that facilitate healthy eating

Promoting healthy lifestyle is a challenging task for many and most of us underestimate the importance of healthy eating. Many people find it difficult to change their lifestyle habits, such as – consumption of alcohol, drugs, smoking, including junk food in their regular diet etc. Lifestyle changes that facilitate healthy eating will show significant decrease in possibilities of chronic diseases.

Eating healthy is not about limiting your food intake, but eliminating all the food you love to eat such as – fried items, sweets, highly processed food, bakery products, oily and spicy food etc. Anyone who wants to change their lifestyle for good health, fitness and well-being should consider healthy eating patterns.

Healthy eating is all about eating in moderation and consuming a variety of food items that are directed to provide all the essential nutrients required by your body. Human body can be said as a complex device created by God, where a number of internal activities take place round the clock to sustain life. In order for the body to perform its day to day activities in a perfect manner, you need to feed your body with essential nutrients. You need to provide your body with appropriate fuel so that it can function at an optimum level.

With busy lifestyle of most of the individuals, this aspect of having healthy eating habits has become quite challenging. Consuming highly processed foods and fast food facilitates ill health in individuals and the end result is chronic diseases. Changing lifestyle habits is one of the best ways to facilitate healthy eating. Always consume foods that enhance the quality of your life and avoid foods that increase the risk of chronic diseases such as cancer, diabetes, heart problem, etc.

You can develop healthy eating habits that bring long term benefits. You can motivate yourself and evaluate your food choice and physical activities. The below lifestyle habits facilitate healthy eating –

1. Making a grocery list and sticking to it
2. Eating breakfast without fail
3. Staying away from deprivation
4. Listening to what your body is saying
5. Access fruits and vegetables on a regular basis
6. Choose wisely, when you dine out
7. Read the food labels, if you are buying processed food.

8. Enjoy whatever you eat. Don't eat just for the sake of satisfying your hunger
9. watch the size of your portion and take it step by step
10. Eat your favorite food carefully

Lifestyle habits that hinder healthy eating

Research shows that people want to be healthy, but don't know how to do so. Hectic lifestyle and busy schedules are hindering healthy eating habits. In today's competitive world, both men and women tend to live in a stressful environment that interferes with healthy eating opportunities. Over time, their stress levels add up to have great impact on their health. Apart from stress, there are a number of lifestyle habits that hinder healthy eating habits and are described as below -

Alcohol

Many people have the habit of drinking and they enjoy it without any problems. Drinking heavily for a long period can have serious consequences like – chronic diseases, spoiled relationships, violence, accidents and even crime.

The recognized immediate effects of consuming alcohol are vomiting and nausea, headache, giddiness, etc. It may effect in a number of other ways and cause brain damage, increased blood pressure, mouth cancer, lung infections, fatty liver, stomach ulcer, inflammation of pancreas, chronic kidney disease, infertility, weight gain, reduced sexual and mental health and many more.

These are not only the ill effects of long term use because even a small amount of alcohol can affect the body. When you consume alcohol, it is absorbed into your blood stream and is passed through different organs. Over time, an individual will be dependent on alcohol physically and mentally. It will become very difficult to gain control and can be life threatening.

Smoking

Smoking is one of the bad habits that not only spoils your life, but also the life of people around you. There is no safe way to smoke. Replacing your cigar with hookah or pipe won't help you in any way. When a cigarette is burnt, it generates more than 7,000 chemicals that are poisonous and can even cause cancer. Cigars have high level of toxins, carcinogens and nicotine that reaches brain in seconds and turns into a habit.

The ill effects of smoking include macular degeneration, poor eye sight, cataract, weak sense of taste and smell, etc. It also damages the respiratory system, cardiovascular system, skin, hair, nails, digestive system and the reproductive system. Some of the dangerous chemicals found in cigarette are tar, carbon mono-oxide, hydrogen cyanide, oxidizing chemicals, metals and radio active compounds.

A lifetime smoker is at a higher risk of developing a broad range of diseases such as bronchitis, liver, ovary and cervix disease, hip fracture, osteoporosis, poor blood circulation in body, ulcers in digestive system, emphysema and many more. Smoking effects and hams almost all the organs of body.

Recreational Drugs Like Marijuana

Drugs are chemicals that can affect human body in various ways. It can be entered into your body through inhalation, injection and ingestion. The method of how it enters the body has a great impact on the health condition of the individual. For example- drugs that are injected into the blood stream have immediate effect. On the contrary, drugs that are ingested pass through digestive system and will not affect the body immediately.

Most of the abused drugs target the brain directly or indirectly by flooding the circuit with a component called 'dopamine' that regulates the movements, emotions, motivation, cognition and feelings of pleasure. When drugs enter into brain, they can change the way your brain performs and lead to compulsive usage. The impact of drug usage is far-reaching and has a negative impact on each and every organ of the body.

Drug use can weaken the immune system of your body and increase your risk of cardiovascular conditions. It may also cause nausea, vomiting, increased liver functioning, stroke, brain damage, increase in body temperature, dramatic fluctuations in appetite and many more. In short, misuse of drugs can be very harmful in short term as well as long term.

How the above habits hinder healthy eating?

All the above bad habits are associated with appetite suppression. Some people consider the above habits as weight-loss tools. On the contrary – smoking, drug misuse and alcohol consumption are related to an increased food intake and severe obesity. Most of the people who have the above habits are reluctant to change their lifestyle and habits because of the concerns of weight gain. In a recent study, it was found that drinking alcohol not only results in chronic health problems; but also has a great impact on the dietary habits.

The influence of alcohol on diet may depend on the amount of alcohol that is being consumed by the individual. It is likely that people who indulge in consuming alcohol may be careless with their eating habits, which will eventually increase their health risk. Moreover, alcohol has a tendency to replace calories from healthy foods that provide nutrition, which leads to a number of nutritional deficiencies.

The bottom line is - making healthy lifestyle changes not only keeps you from chronic health diseases; but also improves your overall health. What you do for yourself is much more important than what medicines can do for you.

Chapter 5
What is the best time to eat your meals?

Even though we have learnt about the right time to eat in childhood in our school lessons, we tend to forget those important lessons conveniently as we get busy with our hectic life. The busy schedule does not permit us to stick to the right eating schedule. However, it is very important to know and follow the right time to eat and to avoid delaying meals. Here are some of the frequently asked questions about what is the best time to have your meals:

> ➤ *Should I eat only when I am hungry?*
> Remember, as a child you ate when you were hungry and stopped eating when your hunger was satiated. As you grew older, this simple rule of

eating becomes distorted by opinions and controversies about how much to eat and when.

"The more you stress, the worse the problem gets", explains Caryn Honig, a professional nutritionist. Her advice is to take cues from your body to understand when you are hungry. Feelings of fatigue and irritability will urge you to eat while those of fullness and pleasant feelings of being satiated will let you know that you are done eating.

➤ *How can I understand my hunger and eating patterns?*
If you are a novice when it comes to recognizing your hungers cues and are unable to figure out when to eat, then note the following explanation. The lack of food can manifest itself in ways that will hamper your normal activity levels by making you feel weak, dizzy and irritable. These unpleasant sensations are indications of hunger; your body is letting you know that you need to eat.

Caryn Honig's advice is to learn to recognize your eating patterns by identifying when you are hungry and understanding when you have eaten enough. You should rate your hunger on a scale of 1 to 10 where 1 is starvation, 2 is very hungry, 3-4 is normal, 6-7 is you can still eat and 8-9 is feeling full with ten at *miserable full*.

Use this scale to analyze and maintain normalcy in your eating patterns. It will help you avoid fatigue from not eating. If you are on a diet, extreme hunger can be followed by overeating afterwards.

> ➢ *I have heard that one should avoid eating after dinner. Is this true?*
You may have grown up hearing the proverb, *eat breakfast like a king, lunch like a prince and dinner like a pauper.* These words of caution were spoken by the well-known American nutritionist, Adele Davis, years ago when it was believed that eating late could cause a range of health problems starting from weight gain to heart burn.

However, the tide of time has diminished the cautionary note of these words as today a calorie is a calorie irrespective of *when* the body intakes it. Your daily calorie intake can be taken in one sitting *or* spread over a number of meals. It all adds up to one single value!

Adjusting your food habits around your daily schedule and bodily requirements creates a framework for timing your meals. If you think a small snack will help you sleep, then you should have it. However, not eating after dinner is good advice for people who are diabetic or obese.

➤ *How can I avoid snacking in front of the television*
Many well known proponents of healthy eating believe that late night eating can end up in a binge sitting in front of the television. Let's say that you are taking in a late night movie and you begin to hanker for snacks. It can begin with the bowl of popcorn and end in a tub of ice-cream! If you are at risk for *binging in front of the telly*, either stop keeping these ready to eat snacks in the kitchen or stop watching the late night shows.

➤ *What is the ideal time gap between dinner and breakfast?*
Given that no two people follow the exact same daily schedule, you can eat your dinner whenever you like and the same goes for breakfast. What

most nutritionists agree on is that you have flexibility to adjust the timings between you first meal in the morning and the last meal of the day. However, whatever time you select, make sure you stick to it on a daily basis and avoid too wide variations in your meal times.

As people are prone to eating meals at specific times, a gap of eight to twelve hours in between dinner and breakfast is automatically created. This gap is considered to be healthy as it gives your body sufficient time to carry out the process of assimilation.

➢ *Is there an example timetable for meals?*
Using a 3-hour gap between meals, an example timetable can be as follows. Eat your morning meal at 6 am and a small snack at 9 am; then lunch can be at noon and dinner at 6pm with a small tea time snack in between. If you are hungry before bedtime, have a small snack at 9 pm.

This timetable should be personalized as per your needs leaving a gap of three to four hours between meals. Keeping a fixed time for your daily meals is a way to inculcate healthy eating as you are able to schedule your day's activities accordingly - giving yourself sufficient time to enjoy your meals.

> *What is the ideal time to have your first morning meal?*
Nutritionists advise eating within an hour of waking up to avoid hunger pangs which may lead to overeating later. When you wake up in the morning, your body has been fasting for the last 8 to 12 hours depending upon the time of your last meal. Eating a tiny snack in the first hour breaks the fast reducing cravings at the breakfast table.

> *How long before bedtime should I eat dinner?*
Most nutritionists agree that eating at least three hours before dinner is a sign of healthy eating. There are some proven problems with eating dinner and going off to sleep immediately afterwards.

If you are a diabetic, going off to sleep immediately after your last major meal that had high sugar levels is not recommended. Also, lying down after a large meal can cause heartburn and acid reflux which you can avoid by eating a few hours before you sleep. If you are working late and the last meal has been four to five hours before, then have a small snack before bedtime.

Studies have shown that if you are obese, eating a low calorie dinner helps you lose more weight than those who eat a high calorie dinner even when the total daily calorie intake for the two groups is the *same.* This indicates that the closer you are to your bedtime, the lesser the number of calories you should intake bearing in mind several factors like age, weight and your ability to digest food whilst asleep.

➢ *I workout for fitness. Should I time my meals around a workout?*
Exercising and eating are two sides of the same coin, which means that you need to eat when you workout. Working out on an empty stomach can lead to dizziness and fatigue. Also, you may feel a lack of energy to begin the workout. A small snack taken 30 minutes before you workout can raise your energy levels and get your metabolism going.

If you workout early mornings, consider eating a light breakfast first to avoid a drop in sugar levels and feelings of weakness from exercising on an empty stomach. Wait for at least an hour after a light breakfast before you workout.

It takes a while to digest the food in your stomach. Therefore exercising right after a meal can make you feel heavy and slow you down. If you choose to eat a large breakfast; wait for about three to four hours before you workout. After a small meal, wait for about two to three hours.

If you workout later in the day, coincide your workout with a major meal time. Exercising will make you hungry and if you eat a proper meal afterwards, then you will be able to satisfy your hunger without resorting to snacking. So timing the end of your workout to coincide with the time of a major meal will help you to keep on schedule to eating healthy!

> *Healthy eating reduces sleep disturbances. Is this true?*
Falling asleep is a problem for many people, especially the elderly. Before you come to any conclusions regarding insomnia and medicines, take a long hard look at your meal schedules and the types of food you are eating before bedtime. If you are going to bed with hunger pangs and a rumbling tummy is keeping you awake, then it is

not surprising that you are not able to sleep. An empty stomach can cause a host of other issues. You should eat a healthy snack before going to bed.

On the other hand; going to bed soon after eating a very rich meal can cause heartburn and prevent you from falling asleep. To prevent these situations eat well before bedtime giving yourself enough time to digest your food.

Hopefully, this will clear all your doubts about when to eat. It is very important to have a fixed schedule of the day for eating as it helps the body to set its own biological clock for digesting the food. This helps to optimize the functions of the digestive organs like secreting juices and regularizing bowel movements thereby ensuring you have no troubles like indigestion, constipation, flatulence, etc.

Chapter 6
Nutrients: How to get the essential nutrients for our body?

For adults, above fifty nutrients are essential for the functions and repair of the body tissues. Adopting healthy eating habits would therefore be beneficial for the mental and physical wellness in aging adults. Providing your body with essential nutrients will help you remain mentally sharp and physically fit and also increase your natural immunity to illnesses and diseases. It will also improve your self-confidence thereby allowing you to be more successful in your professional and personal life.

We eat the food not the nutrients!

If the word nutrients bring forth images of vitamin pills, powders and unappetizing looking cans and jars then you are wrong. These are prescribed to root out nutritional deficiencies in people who need them. For the majority of people, a balanced diet is the source of all the nutrients the body needs to function normally.

The food you intake is broken down as it travels through your digestive system by special chemicals (enzymes and acids) present in the body. These chemicals help break down food into simple components that can be readily absorbed by the tissues. We know these processes as digestion, absorption and assimilation.

Why do you need nutrients?

Your bodily functions depend completely on the nutrients you provide via the foods you intake. The saying, *you are what you eat* makes sense. When you eat a balanced diet your tissues receive the right amounts of nutrients they need. The organs function well and you tend to feel emotionally balanced. These are not casual rewards of eating well; but are also the vital requirements for you to lead a balanced and healthy life.

When do nutrients become essential to the human body?

As you grow older, your calorie requirements lessen making it essential that you make every calorie count by packing it with the nutrients your body requires.

After you cross 50, your calorie requirements begin to decline. For women, the daily required calories decrease to levels between 1600 and 2000 depending on the activity level.

For older men, the daily calorie requirement lies between 2000 and 2800, the higher calorie counts being for those who lead very active lives.

Research has shown that as you age the ability of your body to absorb certain nutrients become less efficient. It is important to keep track of your intake of Vitamin B12, Folic Acid and Calcium after you cross 50. It's a good idea to add foods rich in these nutrients to your diet progressively as you get older.

What are the main groups of nutrients essential for the body?

All the foods you eat can be distributed over six main classes of nutrients, known as carbohydrates, fats, proteins, vitamins, minerals and water.

Carbohydrates

Carbohydrates provide the bulk of the energy requirements of the body. Without carbohydrate, body functions would not be possible. The main sources of carbohydrates are sugars and starches. Sugar is a ready-to-use source of energy from sugar-based products like jams and jellies that can be absorbed and used by the body instantly. Starches are complex carbs that need to be broken down before the body can use them. Foods that contain starch are potatoes, cereals and pasta. Carbohydrates that the body gets from whole grains and fruits also contain fiber that can prevent heart attacks and ease digestion.

Fats

Fats are composed of carbon, oxygen and hydrogen. Saturated fats contained in oils that are a medium of frying and cooking should be minimal. Fats are a source of energy and help in the absorption of fat-soluble vitamins like A, D, E and K. Fats should be consumed via healthy rich Omega-3 sources like fish and nuts. Saturated fats that come from fatty meats and the full fat dairy products should be avoided.

Proteins

Proteins are the main building blocks of the body responsible for the growth and repair of muscles, skin and hair. Proteins can be broken down in to complex amino acid molecules that are the basic components of our body's tissues. A diet must have at least 10 to 35 percent protein for good health. This nutrient can be found in low fat dairy, eggs, peas, beans and lean meat.

Vitamins

Your body requires essential vitamins to stay healthy and prevent diseases. For example; Vitamin A is good for the eyes, skin and for hair growth. Vitamin D helps in calcium absorption by the tissues of the bone and teeth, while Vitamin C helps fight infections. Citrus fruits, strawberries and bell peppers are rich sources of vitamins.

Minerals

Minerals are inorganic substances required in various quantities by the body. Sodium, Calcium and Potassium are required along with traces of fluorine and zinc. Sodium is essential for maintaining the body's fluid levels and its daily intake should be less than 2400 milligram. Potassium helps lower the blood pressure. Calcium is important for maintaining bone density. Iron is another mineral required in small amounts by the body. Citrus fruits like banana are a good source of minerals.

Water

All the water you drink gives you zero energy. Yet, water is essential for you to remain hydrated and for your body to carry out its routine functions. It helps to maintain body temperature (homeostasis), break down the food we eat and carry waste products out of the body. A healthy body needs between 2 to 3 liters of water daily.

Framework of a balanced diet

A diet that provides nutrients from all the six major groups in their correct proportion is said to be a balanced diet. The food pyramid is an example of a framework that can be used to plan meals.

It clearly illustrates in the form of a triangle the major type of foods that you need to consume for fitness and health. The base of the triangle is where most of the food you eat should originate; about 60 to 70 percent constitute your intake of carbs and unsaturated fats rich in Omega-3. As you move up the triangle toward the tip, the food items begin to represent proteins sourced from dairy and meats forming about 30 to 40 percent of your diet. The consumption of saturated fats like cooking oils and butter should be minimized.

The end result of a nutritious diet is manifold: higher mental alacrity as the brain is receiving the nutrients necessary for tissue growth; longevity due to the lowered risk from chronic diseases and a sense of well being that makes you feel happy.

Taking nutrients in the form of supplements

Supplements can be used to provide many of the nutrients necessary for the body. However, as the supplements do not contain the required bulk from fiber, the body suffers from the lack of it. Food containing large amounts of fiber helps in keeping the digestion process smooth and efficient.

Basic tips for maintaining a healthy diet

- Reduce salt, keep your salt intake under 2400 milligram
  - High sodium diet can increase blood pressure
- Avoid foods with added sugar
  - These can be found in processed foods and sweetened drinks
  - Check the label before you buy.
- Do not eat polished grains and refined sugar

- o These constitute bad carbs that can fluctuate your sugar levels
  - o Polished grains do not contain the nutrients as they are removed during their processing.
- Eat foods having five different colors on your plate
  - o This is a sign of eating nutritious foods
- Transition from frying to steaming your food
  - o Frying adds saturated fats to your foods which you don't want

Avoiding malnutrition

It is often seen that well-fed people over the age of 50 suffer from malnutrition. This is not surprising as the foods they are eating are not nutritious enough to provide an adequate amount of nutrients the body needs for functioning normally. This can lead to a series of health issues like fatigue and depression, heart disease, lung disease, anemia, lowered immunity and skin problems amongst others.

Preventing malnutrition as you age should be of concern. Eat from a variety of foods having five different colors and flavors and with others. Prepare colorful meals along with others and eat together. You need to improve your food intake by snacking between meals. In extreme case consult your doctor.

There are a few more things to consider for your general well-being. You need to be careful about weight gain and obesity by exercising regularly to remain fit. Your diet is a key to good health; so make sure that all food groups are represented in your meals. Keep in mind that the food triangle is a useful framework. When you use it as a guide, you are ensured that you are eating right. However, as no two people are the same, you have the freedom to select the foods you prefer to create a balanced meal for yourself.

It is a blessing that life's pleasures come in all shapes and sizes and not in the shape of wholesome nutrients! It is far nicer to bite into a juicy citrus fruit than take a vitamin C tablet. The colors of mother earth are manifested in the foods we grow in the soil and eat. Your body gives you the freedom to choose and fill your plates with as many colors as you fancy. This is the essence of wellbeing and the celebration of life in an innocuous way!

Chapter 7
Conclusion

The following FAQ further tests your knowledge of healthy eating. You can also use it to briefly review the information presented above for your benefit.

1. **Healthy eating means giving up all the things you love?**

    • This is not true. If you have a sweet tooth for desserts and fried foods, you should not try to stop eating them immediately as a one time attempt to become totally health conscious. It is possible that the cravings will get you back to eating these food items again. Instead, phase them out gradually from your meals and snack times by eating smaller and smaller portions and less often.

- Sometimes, replacing fatty deserts with their less harmful counterparts can be a smart move. For example; plain milk chocolate is said to be good for the heart and libido. Dark chocolate contains disease fighting flavonoids and antioxidants good for lowering cholesterol.

2. Poor diet and lack of exercise can cause heart disease?

- Yes, a diet containing large quantities of bad carbohydrates, animal fats, trans-fats and saturated fats places a person at the risk for heart disease, cholesterol and obesity. A sedentary lifestyle indicates that most of the calories received from a poor diet is not used by the body; but gets converted to unwanted fats worsening the problem.

- Sometimes dieters replace the regular versions of their food items with non-fat, fat-free and sugar-free foods. One has to be careful that the item is truly what it says it is by learning to read the nutrition labels on these food items.

- For example a label that says trans fat-free may still contain saturated fats, which is not good for the heart. Further 0 trans fat-free on labels can have as much as legally allowed 0.5 amounts of trans fat per serving, which is not exactly fat-free.

- Also 0 cholesterol-free labels are allowed so long as the food item contains no more than 2mg of cholesterol and less than 2 grams of saturated fats per serving. Taken in large quantities saturated fats and trans fats raise LDL - bad cholesterol levels placing one at risk for heart disease. Coconut and palm oils contain saturated fats and margarine (sticks) and shortening used by bakeries contain trans fats and should be avoided.

3. Should women take more dairy products?

- Aging women need to raise their intake of calcium to maintain a healthy skeleton and reduce their risk of osteoporosis and bone fracture. Good source of calcium like milk can help reduce the risk of osteoporosis.

- Mayo Clinic suggests taking Vitamin D to help aid calcium absorption by the body from the foods you eat.

4. Does potassium found in banana help to lower blood pressure?

- That is true. Minerals are an important group of nutrients required by your body and help prevent diseases. Potassium not only lowers blood pressure; but is good for your muscles and nerves too. Other sources of potassium are milk, potatoes, sweet potatoes, avocado and legumes.

5. Lowering the intake of sugar, salt and saturated fats supports healthy eating?

- Sugar is considered as bad carbs as it raises blood sugar levels and is the chief cause of obesity raising your exposure to type 2diabetes, heart disease, arthritis and certain types of cancers. Minimizing sugar intake via sweetened drinks and processed foods would be a healthy move.

- Sodium causes heart disease and therefore saying no to salt would be a positive move toward a healthy heart.

- Saturated fats exist in margarine sticks and shortening that is widely used in baking. Taking some time to read the labels on baked goods packages can help you move to their healthier counterparts having less salts, sugars and saturated fats.

6. Eating disorders have nothing to do with your mental health?

- This is not true. Eating disorder is related to food habits that prevent you from eating a balanced diet, which provide all the key nutrients to the body. Eating well and exercising help you prevent diseases like dementia and Alzheimer's.

- On a more positive note, when you eat well your body is able to provide the energy required for you to carry out your daily activities. Your feeling of well-being lifts your spirits making you happy and stress-free.

7. **Planning your grocery before you reach the store is a waste of time?**

- This is not true. Making a list of essential ingredients you need to purchase from the grocery for the meals you plan to make promotes the effort you make toward eating healthy. Arriving at the grocery without a planned list would be a waste of time as you would end up buying ingredients arbitrarily.

8. **You should not eat unless you are hungry. True or false?**

- True. Your body has its own metabolic cycle and eating when you are hungry is a good sign that you are listening to the hunger cues from your body. However, you should take care to eat adequately at meal times.

- If you have fixed meal times, then you should adjust them suitably such that you can eat when you are hungry.

9. Diet and exercise can help you remain mentally sharp as you age?

- Your diet is a very important aspect and the key to mental wellness. When you eat well, you provide your body with the essential nutrients necessary for it to carry out its functions. Exercise helps your blood circulation supply oxygen and nutrients to all parts of the body, remove waste products and strengthen your skeletal muscles. All of this helps to keep you physically fit and mentally alert as you age.

10. Is it possible for you to suffer from malnutrition?

- Yes. Even well-fed people can suffer from malnutrition. In order to avoid nutritional deficiencies, you must eat suitably from the following food groups
  - Fruits and vegetable
  - Whole grains
  - Legumes, omega-3 fatty foods like fish
  - Lean meat and dairy

How well you fare in your journey toward healthy eating depends entirely upon you. Slowly changing your eating habits to turn more and more toward healthy eating is a necessity and a challenge well worth taking.

Good Luck!

Finally, if you enjoyed this book or found it useful in some way, I would like to ask you for a favor. Would you be kind enough **to leave a review** for this book? It would be appreciated greatly!

Thank you very much.

Dominique Kaneza, Author

Bonus:

Join the exclusive mailing list and receive a FREE Ebook

www.tmapublishing.com

Also from author:

AGING BACKWARDS: Prevent Premature Aging and Look
10 Years Younger!:
How To Stay Young and Healthy After Menopause

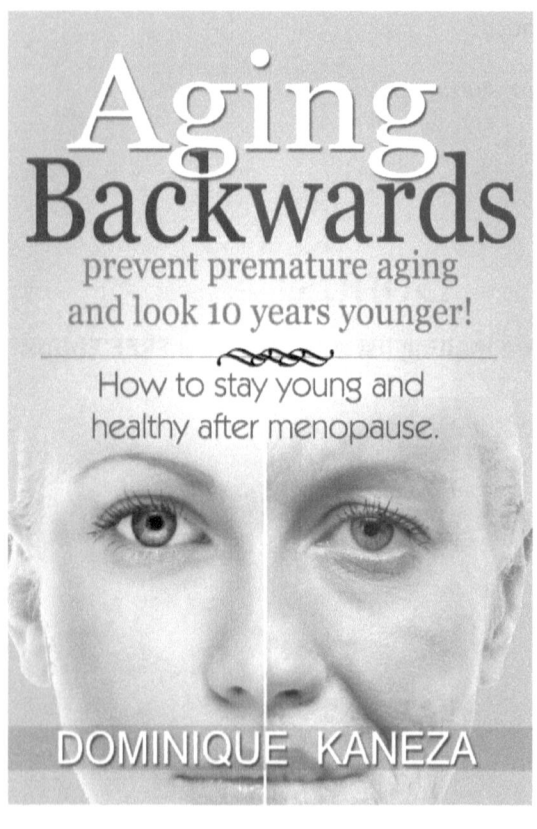